Natural Remedies
for Health, Beauty and Home

EPSOM SALT

Josephine Simon

Copyrights

Disclaimer and Terms of Use

ISBN: 978-1542752220

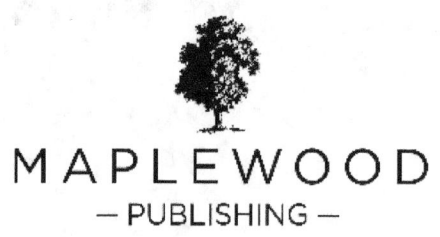

MAPLEWOOD
— PUBLISHING —

Contents

Introduction

Epsom Salt has been the talk of the town for some time, especially lately, after none other than Victoria Bekham and Gwyneth Paltrow attributed their flat stomachs to it. Contestants of "Dancing with the Stars" confessed to using Epsom salt to relieve pain, erase bruises, and recondition their bodies for the next highly-taxing dance round.

For some, Epsom Salt may just be something one would group together with baking soda and borax, possibly. Maybe it would be something between a cleaning agent and a folk remedy. Perhaps it was just Grandma who knew about it but couldn't convince you to try it. But now, you hear about it in news headlines, mom blogs, fashion and beauty magazines, celebrity gossip, and websites on alternative medicine, medical articles, and testimonies from athletes – you name it. Epsom Salt is definitely making a splash. Many swear by its myriad of benefits. It is said to be effective for relieving pain, reducing inflammation, speeding recovery, fighting off the cold and flu, beautifying skin and hair, cleansing, detoxifying, regulating blood pressure, and so much more. Not only does it heal and beautify, it is also has wonderful uses in gardening, pet care, and even in making crafts.

And, to top this all – it's cheap!

This book gives a bit of history and an explanation of the principle behind the use and the beneficial effects of Epsom salt. Here you will find recipes for health, beauty, home, garden, pets, and more. The recipes' uses are written in bold letters above each one. You will find most of the recipes simple and easy to follow.

Epsom salt is actually not a new fad. It has been recognized for its many uses for several centuries. As you turn the pages of this book, you will find many ways to use Epsom salt to heal, perhaps not only the body, but the soul as well. You'll experience firsthand what everyone's raving about!

A Glance Back at How Epsom Salt Was First Discovered

It all started in 1618 in the town of Epsom in Surrey, England. A man named Henry Wicker found some water that his cattle refused to drink. He tasted the bitter water and was the first to experience its benefits. Word began to spread and soon, people from all over England and Europe came to visit Epsom to avail of the water's healing qualities. The town of Epsom soon became a famous place to visit.

The waters' healing properties came from the crystals that could be scraped from the bottom of the wells. It was a certain Nehemiah Grew who named the crystals "Epsom Salts" in 1695. It was also discovered that these salts could be found in caves and mines. Epsom salt now comes from different sources but still carries the name of the town where it all began.

What Is Epsom Salt?

Its name is sometimes in the plural – Epsom *Salts*. It is referred to as a salt or *salts* even though it isn't the same as the salt (sodium chloride) that we use for cooking, and neither does it consist of many "salts." It is a mineral compound that looks a lot like ordinary table salt.

The chemical name for Epsom Salt is Magnesium Sulfate. The more familiar or household form is the heptahydrate. It is referred to as an inorganic salt, a neutral chemical compound that is soluble in water. From its formula, $MgSO_4$ (or $MgSO_4 \cdot 7H_2O$ in its more common form), you see that it contains Magnesium, Sulfur, and Oxygen. The magnesium in Epsom Salt may be the major reason behind all its amazing properties.

Magnesium holds the key

Magnesium is one of the most important minerals needed by the body. It is an essential macro-mineral. This means that it cannot be manufactured by the human body and that it is needed in large amounts. Our bodies require at least 320 mg of it every day. Some experts believe that the recommended daily allowance (RDA) for magnesium should be doubled.

Magnesium is responsible for two very important functions at the cellular level – producing energy and creating new cells. About 300 biological functions in the human body require magnesium. A shortage of it would affect several of the body's functions, resulting in severe illness, pain, and incapacity. The lack of it would speed up the aging process, and result in all kinds of undesirable symptoms related to the muscular, neurological, metabolic, and cardiovascular systems of the body.

Magnesium is important to our brain, muscles, heart, and blood vessels. High blood pressure, diabetes, asthma, osteoporosis, and heart disease often result from magnesium deficiency. The largest reserves of this mineral are found in the heart. There has been much emphasis on the importance of calcium in the body without emphasizing the need to balance it with magnesium. A person with a magnesium deficiency could suffer a heart attack even if he were not deficient in calcium.

Even with a healthy diet, we may still not be getting enough magnesium. This is because it has already been depleted from the soil due to overcropping and the use of strong chemical fertilizers. Thus, plants are also lacking in this mineral. The effects of deficiency in this important mineral can be avoided by taking supplements. This is especially important for adults because the body's absorption of magnesium declines with age.

Although a bit controversial and still not completely explained scientifically, magnesium is said to enter the body through the skin. Epsom salt baths are recommended as a way for the body to absorb the mineral and correct any deficiency. People who have tried Epsom salt baths swear to have found healing and relief from pain, sleeplessness, depression, PMS, and other health issues related to magnesium deficiency.

Epsom salt is taken internally more as a laxative than as a magnesium supplement.

A bit about sulfates

To give credit where due, the role of sulfate in the overall effect of Epsom salt should not be overlooked. Sulfate, like magnesium, is also important in several of the body's biological processes and is also absorbed through the skin. It improves absorption of other nutrients and helps in flushing out toxins from the body. It plays a major role in the formation of proteins in the joints, a deficiency of which would result in rheumatoid arthritis. It initiates the chain reaction of enzymes involved in the digestive process.

Mucin proteins, which are important in preventing the guts from sticking as well as to filter out toxins attempting to enter the digestive tract, cannot be formed without sulfate. Another one of its crucial responsibilities involves the formation of brain tissue and maintenance of neurons. Sulfate is also noted for its action against migraines.

Health Benefits in a Nutshell

Here are the top 10 health benefits from Epsom salt:
1. Relieves pain and cramping
2. Relaxes the body and soothes the nerves
3. Regulates blood pressure
4. Flushes out toxins

5. Regulates blood sugar
6. Improves muscle and nerve function
7. Improves blood circulation
8. Contributes to weight loss
9. Reduces the risk of heart attacks
10. Relieves constipation

Uses

The versatility of Epsom salt is evident in the range and diversity of its uses.

For Health
1. Bath salt for soaking to relieve stress, muscle pain, sprains, and soreness, as well as for injury prevention and faster healing
2. After-working out ice bath
3. Oral laxative
4. Intravenous medicine for seizures
5. Nebulizer treatment for asthma
6. Gall bladder and liver flush
7. Gout remedy
8. Detoxifier
9. Eyewash
10. Migraine remedy
11. Hangover remedy
12. Jet lag remedy
13. Sleep aid

14. Treatment for bug bites, sunburn, and irritated skin
15. Treatment for bee sting and poison ivy irritation
16. Treatment for nail and toe fungus
17. Treatment for foot odor
18. Bruise treatment
19. Splinter remover
20. Tooth Whitener and Cleaner
21. Weight loss aid

For Beauty

1. Facial wash
2. Hand wash
3. Exfoliant for removing rough, dry and callused skin
4. Treatment and smoothener for dry lips
5. Hair clarifier and volumizer
6. Rejuvenating skin mask
7. Anti-frizz
8. Heat protection for hair
9. Blackhead remover

For the home

1. Tile and grout cleaner
2. Cookware cleaner
3. Detergent residue remover
4. Fabric softener
5. Battery booster

For the garden
1. Fertilizer and plant supplement
2. Flowering agent
3. Bug repellent
4. Weed killer
5. Slug Deterrent

For pets
1. Nail abscess infection remedy
2. Pet shampoo and whitener
3. Itch reliever

Others
1. Fake snow and frost décor
2. No-Slip Surface
3. Raccoon repellent

Just a few precautions

Epsom salt is generally considered to be mild and very safe to use, but as with any supplement or medication, it's always best to take precautions.

People who are dehydrated or who have open cuts or burns on their skin should not use the Epsom salt bath.

Pregnant women and people with a weak heart or kidney problems must consult a doctor first.

People with known allergies to the components of Epsom salt should not use it. Symptoms of allergy are itching, hives, swelling of the lips, tongue or any part of the face, difficulty breathing, and chest tightness. Look out also for faintness, dizziness, drowsiness, sweating, muscle paralysis, or irregular heartbeat.

When used as a laxative, follow the directions in the packaging. What may be safe for some may be toxic for others. Discontinue use if you experience any swelling, flushing, nausea, dizziness, or lower back pain after ingesting. These are signs of magnesium overdose and can be life-threatening.

Soaking in an Epsom salt bath may aggravate a very dry skin condition.

Though very rare, some infections caused by fungi and staphylococcus can be worsened by soaking in hot water. This could be the case if you notice no positive changes to an infected cut or wound even after soaking in Epsom salt. Normally, soaking gives rapid relief to pain and inflammation in infected cuts.

Not All Epsom Salt Is Created Equal

Not all Epsom salt is safe for ingestion. There is Epsom Salt for Agricultural use and those for personal use. Look for the label that says United States Pharmaceutical Grade or "USP" grade. This may also be labeled "Food Grade," meaning that your Epsom salt is pure and safe for human use. USP grade meets the requirements of the US Food and Drug Administration or FDA.

"Technical Grade," also called "Agricultural Grade" or "Industrial Grade," may contain some impurities because inspection for this grade is not as stringent or regular as that for USP. There is also other, cheaper Epsom salts from different sources, but these are not graded and are more likely to contain impurities or even some heavy metals.

Recipes for Health

In the introduction, the health benefits of Epsom salt are discussed, and its many possible uses for health are enumerated. Now, it's time to try out some tried-and-tested recipes that have helped so many people find success in their fight against pain, fatigue, debilitation, and weariness. Join the many who have conquered illnesses using a cheap, readily available resource. Most treatments using Epsom salt are usually very simple. No fancy equipment or ingredients needed. Follow these recipes as you embark on a journey that will never make you look back.

For Muscle Pain, Bruises, Colds and Flu, Itching, Sleep Difficulties, Stress, and Jetlag

Basic Epsom Salt Bath

Soaking in an Epsom salt bath will make you experience its health benefits. Many feel renewed, refreshed, and invigorated after trying it. You will feel relief from muscle pain, soreness, and stiffness. After the bath, you will have a restful sleep.

Dosages may vary depending on the brand, source, grade, or the purpose of the treatment. There are many variations to the Epsom Salt Bath to accommodate different needs or preferences. Always read the instructions in the packaging.

The standard measures based on body weight are as follows:

For children under 60 lbs	1/2 cup of Epsom salt
For individuals weighing 60-100 lbs	1 cup of Epsom salt
For individuals weighing 100-150 lbs	1 1/2 cup of Epsom salt
For individuals weighing 150-200 lbs	2 cups of Epsom salt

Add ½ cup more for each additional 50 lbs in weight.

Instructions:
1. Dissolve the Epsom salt by adding it while running the bath.
2. Soak for at least 12 minutes.

Moisturizing Epsom Salt Bath

For a standard-sized bathtub, you'll need:

2 cups Epsom salt for adults weighing between 150-200 lbs.
Adjust the quantity according to the table.
Warm water (not too hot; pleasant to the touch)
½ cup olive or baby oil, optional
Eucalyptus or lavender oils, optional
1-4 tablespoons ginger or cayenne, optional

For a large-sized bathtub, use
3-4 cups Epsom salt

Instructions:
1. Add the Epsom salt while filling the tub to thoroughly dissolve crystals. Add baby or olive oils for to soften skin; a few drops lavender oil for a more relaxing effect or eucalyptus oil for an invigorating scent; cayenne or ginger to enhance sweating (optional).
2. Soak for at least 12 minutes, making sure that affected part is fully submerged.
3. Relax and rest for about 2 hours after soaking.

To detox, repeat twice a week.
Do not use bath soap as this will interfere with the action of the Epsom salt.

Cayenne and ginger add heat to promote sweating. Caution is advised in adding herbs and oils as these may cause skin irritation or allergic reactions.

Ideally, filtered water without toxins and impurities should be used to maximize the detox effect.

NOTE: For those with arthritis, movement after soaking is needed to prevent congestion of the joints.

For Muscle Pain, Splinters, and Poison Ivy Irritation

Cold Compress

You'll need:
2-4 tablespoons Epsom salt
1-2 cups cold water

Instructions:
1. Mix the Epsom salt and water together.
2. Soak a clean piece of cotton cloth or face towel in the solution. Gently squeeze out any excess.
3. Apply to affected area. Repeat as needed.
4. For splinters: You might need to use tweezers to pull out splinters that have been drawn to the skin surface.

For Muscle Pain

Warm Compress

You'll need:
1 cup Epsom salt
2 gallons of warm water

Instructions:

1. Combine Epsom salt and water in a pot or basin.
2. Soak a clean cotton cloth or face towel in the solution. Gently squeeze off any excess.
3. Apply on affected area until it cools down.
4. Repeat.

For Muscle Pain, Splinters, and Skin Inflammation

Healing Paste

You'll need:

1 teaspoon Epsom salt
1 cup hot water

Instructions:

1. Stir Epsom salt in water until dissolved.
2. Refrigerate solution for 20 minutes.
3. Clean affected area. Pat dry.
4. Apply paste.

For Sore, Aching, or Smelly Feet

Epsom Salt Footbath 1

You'll need:
1 cup Epsom salt
Warm water

Instructions:
1. Fill a footbath or basin with warm water.
2. Pour in Epsom salt.
3. Soak feet.

For Poor Blood Circulation, Pain, and Inflammation

Epsom Salt Footbath 2

You'll need:
½ cup Epsom salt
1 gallon hot water (16 cups), as tolerable

Instructions:
1. Dissolve Epsom salt in water. Test hotness before soaking.
2. Soak feet for 10 minutes, 2-3 times a week.

For Toenail Fungus

Footbath for Toenail Fungus

You'll need:
1 cup Epsom salt
Hot water, tolerable enough to immerse feet

Instructions:
1. Dissolve Epsom salt in hot water. Test water before soaking.
2. Soak feet for about 10 minutes, 2 times a day.

For Infections of Superficial Wounds or Cuts

Anti-infection Soak

You'll need:
2 teaspoons Epsom salt
2 cups hot water, as tolerable

Instructions:
1. Dissolve Epsom salt in hot water. Keep in a kettle to maintain heat.
2. Fill a basin with enough solution to immerse affected part.
3. Make sure the heat of solution will not cause scalding. Soak affected part in hot solution.
4. Remove affected part, and add more hot solution.

5. Soak for 6-10 minutes. Do not soak longer than this.
6. Repeat every few hours several times throughout the day.

Note: Soaking the affected part frequently in a day has been observed to be more effective than increasing soaking duration.

For The Common Cold or Flu

Cold Cure

You'll need:
2-3 cups Epsom salt
Hot water, as tolerable, to fill a tub

Instructions:
1. Before preparing the bath, be sure to have 2-3 blankets or large towels within reach. You may also need a timer or alarm clock.
2. Run hot water into bathtub, pouring in Epsom salt to dissolve.
3. Test for water temperature before getting into tub.
4. Soak in the tub, making sure to immerse your whole body. Immersing your head will help clear clogged nasal passages.
5. Soak for about 6 minutes. Get out immediately if your pulse is racing.
6. You must dry yourself off in not more than 1 minute to avoid chills. Quickly wrap yourself in prepared towels or blankets.
7. Lie down and allow your body to sweat for 20-40 minutes.
8. Take a shower, taking care not to get chilled.

9. Drink water to replace lost body fluid.
10. Repeat every 2-3 hours within the day.
11. Rest for a day or two to recover your strength.

For Gout Relief

Soak for Gout

You'll need:
2-3 teaspoons Epsom salt
Basin of hot water, as tolerable

Instructions:
1. Dissolve the Epsom salt in water. Test temperature before soaking affected area.
2. Soak affected joint or foot for 30 minutes.

For Itchy Skin, Bug Bites, and Minor Sunburn

Epsom Salt Spritz

You'll need:
1 tablespoon Epsom salt
½ cup warm water

Instructions:

1. Dissolve Epsom salt in water.
2. Cool to room temperature or a little cooler, if desired.
3. Transfer to spray bottle.
4. Spritz over affected area.

For Muscle Pain, Shoulder Pain, and Skin Inflammation

Shoulder Pain Remedy

You'll need:

1 cup Epsom salt
1 cup lukewarm water

Instructions:

1. Mix Epsom salt and water together.
2. Gently massage over affected area.
3. Rinse off with warm water.
4. You may do this before taking a shower.

For Constipation

Epsom Salt Laxative Solution

You'll need:
1 teaspoon Epsom salt, Food Grade
½ cup (4 ounces) water
1 teaspoon lemon juice (optional)

Instructions:
1. Add Epsom salt to water and stir to dissolve. Add lemon juice to improve taste (optional).
2. Drink.
3. Expect a movement within 30 minutes to 6 hours.

NOTE: Check the packaging of your Epsom salt for exact dosage. Epsom salt is generally safe, but it is best to consult a doctor before using it as a laxative.

For Tooth Stains and Periodontal Disease

Tooth Whitener and Cleaner

You'll need:
2 tablespoons Epsom Salt
1/8 cup water

Instructions:

1. Mix the Epsom salt with water.
2. Use to brush teeth and/or to gargle.

For Weight Loss

Weight Loss and Detox Bath

You'll need:

1-2 cups Epsom salt
1 cup baking soda
2 tablespoons bath oil, optional
Hot water to fill standard size bathtub

Instructions:

1. Run water into tub.
2. Add Epsom salt, baking soda, and oil (optional).
3. Soak in bath for at least 12 minutes (not more than 25 minutes) 3 times a week or every night.
4. Drink a glass of water while soaking in the bath.
5. Should be done along with diet and exercise.

To Flush Out Gallstones

Warning: Do not attempt if you have not had an ultrasound scan to determine the size of your gallstones. Gallstones that are too large may be painful, difficult, and dangerous to dislodge using this method.

Gallstone Flush

You'll need:

12 liters apple juice, preferably from green apples, freshly squeezed or organic

Chamomile Tea, optional

1-2 tablespoons Epsom salt

½ cup extra virgin olive oil, cold-pressed, unrefined

¼ cup lemon juice, freshly squeezed

Instructions:

1. Prep for the flush is done for 5 consecutive days. The flush is done on the 6th day.

For 5 consecutive days

1. Drink 2 liters of apple juice a day.
2. Drink about 5 cups of chamomile tea a day (optional).
3. You should preferably eat a vegetarian diet rich in whole grains, beans, and soy products, avoiding sugar, coffee, ice cold drinks and greasy foods. Do not skip meals and do not eat excessively.

4. You must also drink 6-8 glasses of water a day.

On the 6th day

1. Do not eat anything after lunch.
2. Continue consuming apple juice and tea.
3. At 9:00 PM, drink Epsom salt dissolved in about ½ cup to 1 cup warm water.
4. At 10:00 PM, mix olive oil and lemon juice together and drink with a straw (to prevent the oil from coming in contact with the lips and to minimize having to taste the liquid).
5. Lie down on your right side. Bring your right knee to your chest to drain the olive oil mixture. You must stay in bed and try to sleep.
6. You should pass the stones anytime from 12 midnight to the next day. The stones will be brown or greenish, of various sizes.
7. A dull pain may indicate a dislodged stone. If you think this is the case, repeat the process.

NOTE: Many who have followed this procedure were spared the need to undergo the expensive process of having their gallstones removed by surgery. However, it is always best to consult a doctor.

For Cataracts, Styes and Conjunctivitis

Epsom Salt Eyewash and Warm Compress

You'll need:
1 teaspoon Epsom salt
1 cup hot water

Instructions:
1. Dissolve Epsom salt in water, stirring to dissolve.
2. Allow to cool down until comfortable to touch.
3. Close eyes and pour eyewash over face.
4. Rinse with cool water.
5. FOR CONJUNCTIVITIS: Soak a clean cloth in solution and place for 2-3 minutes over affected eye as warm compress. Rinse. Repeat 2-3 times a week.

Recipes for Beauty

Surprisingly, Epsom salt has been proven to be a cheap alternative to some beauty products. But cheap doesn't mean inferior. The results are just as good, if not better, than using expensive, branded beauty aids. Epsom salt also gives you a health boost as you use it to groom yourself. Without having to spend so much at a spa, you'll enjoy luxurious pampering in your own home. Be healthy inside and beautiful outside!

To Remove Rough, Dead Skin and Calluses

Exfoliating Scrub

You'll need:
Epsom salt
Water
Coconut or olive oil, optional

Instructions:
1. Moisten Epsom salt to make a paste. Add a drop or two of oil (optional).
2. Massage over damp skin.
3. Rinse.

To Gently Exfoliate, Cleanse and Treat Acne

Facial Wash

You'll need:
½ teaspoon Epsom salt
1 dollop of creamy facial cleanser

Instructions:
1. Mix together.
2. Apply on face in circular motions.
3. Rinse off.

Cleansing and Softening for Oily Skin

Face Mask

You'll need:
1 tablespoon Cognac
1 egg
¼ cup non-fat dry milk
2-3 tablespoons lemon juice
½ teaspoon Epsom salt

Instructions:
1. Mix ingredients together.
2. Dampen face.
3. Apply to skin and leave on for 20 minutes.
4. Rinse off.

To Remove Beauty Product Buildup and Greasiness in Hair

Hair Clarifier

You'll need:
1 cup lemon juice
1 cup Epsom salt
1 gallon water

Instructions:
1. Mix together and let stand for 24 hours.
2. Use to rinse hair.

To Treat Limp, Greasy Hair

Hair Volumizer

You'll need:
2 tablespoons Epsom salt
2 tablespoons hair conditioner
Instructions:
1. Combine and apply on hair.
2. Leave on for 20 minutes.
3. Rinse.
4. Use once a week.

To Add Texture and Volume to Hair

Hair Spray

You'll need:
1 cup hot water
½ teaspoon sea salt
1 teaspoon Aloe Vera gel
½ teaspoon hair conditioner
A few drops essential oil of choice (optional)

Instructions:
1. Combine in a 10-ounce size jar. Place lid on jar and shake until contents and salt are dissolved.
2. Transfer to a spray bottle.
3. Spray on damp hair and scrunch for waves.
4. Spray on dry hair for volume.

To Cleanse and Soften Hands

Hand wash

You'll need:
½ cup Epsom salt
½ cup baby oil

Instructions:
1. Mix together.
2. Keep in a container near your sink.

For Deep Exfoliation

Lavender Scrub

You'll need:
2 cups Epsom salt
¼ cup petroleum jelly
A few drops lavender oil

Instructions:
1. Moisten skin under a warm shower for about 5 minutes. Turn off shower.
2. Massage scrub very gently over skin in circular motions.
3. Rinse off. Pat skin dry.

NOTE: Do not use if skin is broken or irritated.

To Soften Dry, Rough Feet

Foot Scrub

You'll need:
1 cup Epsom salt
¼ cup almond, coconut, olive, or baby oil
1 teaspoon liquid castile soap
10-15 drops essential oil of desired scent

Instructions:
1. Mix ingredients together.
2. Store in an airtight container.
3. Use a small amount to scrub feet, hands or body.
4. Rinse.

For Gentle Removal of Blackheads

Blackhead Remover

You'll need:
1 teaspoon Epsom salt
3 drops iodine
½ cup boiling water
Astringent

Instructions:
1. Combine the Epsom salt, iodine, and boiling water.
2. Allow to cool down until comfortable to touch.
3. Saturate a cotton ball and apply on affected area.
4. Repeat 3-4 times, reheating solution if needed.
5. Remove blackheads gently.
6. Apply astringent.

To Treat Dry, Chapped or Cracked Lips

Lip Smoothener

You'll need:
1 teaspoon Epsom salt
2 teaspoons petroleum jelly

Instructions:
1. Combine and rub on lips and then wipe off.

Scented Bath Salts for Later Use or as Gift Idea

Bath Salts

You'll need:
2 cups Epsom salt
Food color
Essential oil of choice

Instructions:
1. Combine and store in airtight jars.
2. To use, add to bath water as desired.
3. Variation: Place the salts in a drawstring cheesecloth pouch to be dipped in the bathwater.

Use Leftover Champagne to Tone Skin and to Detox

Post-Celebration Toning and Detox Bath

You'll need:
1 cup Epsom Salt
1 cup powdered milk
1 cup champagne
1 teaspoon honey, warm
Flower petals, like rose or orchid

Instructions:
1. Add everything while running water into bathtub.
2. Scatter flower petals over water.
3. Soak in, relax, and enjoy.

Recipes for the Home

The use and exposure to harsh or synthetic chemicals can have dangerous effects on the health, not only of everyone in the household, but also on the environment in general. It's a good thing Epsom salt is a gentle, natural, cheap, and effective option for many household uses.

To Clean Tiles

Tile and Grout Cleaner

You'll need:
1 cup Epsom salt
1 cup Dishwashing detergent

Instructions:
1. Combine and use to scrub tiles.
2. Rinse and wipe dry.

To Remove Burnt Food from Pans

Cookware Cleaner

You'll need:
1 teaspoon Epsom salt
Warm water

Instructions:
1. Dissolve the Epsom salt in some warm water. A less dilute solution will give more scouring power.
2. Scrub pans. Rinse.

A Natural Cleaner for Removing Water Stains

Hard Water Stain Scrub

You'll need:
1 cup Epsom salt
½ cup baking soda
¼ cup dishwashing liquid

Instructions:
1. Mix together thoroughly.
2. Make sure surfaces are dry before applying stain scrub.
3. Apply on tiles and bathroom surfaces with a cloth.
4. Leave on for 10 minutes.

5. Scrub again.
6. Rinse off with warm water.
7. Wipe surfaces dry to prevent new water stains from forming.

Eco-Friendly Laundry Detergent for a Soft, Clean Wash

Laundry Detergent

You'll need:
1 12-ounce box borax
1 4-pound box baking soda
4 pounds Epsom salt
3 bars pure castile soap, grated

Instructions:
1. Mix together thoroughly.
2. Use about 1 tablespoon for small loads and 2 tablespoons for large loads. Fabric softener is not needed.

NOTE: Epsom salt is especially helpful when using hard water as it breaks down the minerals in the water.

For Soft, Fluffy and Fresh-Smelling Clothes

Fabric Softener

You'll need:
1 cup Epsom salt
10 drops essential oil of choice

Instructions:
1. Mix together thoroughly and store in a jar.
2. Use ¼ cup for regular loads and 1/3 cup for large loads.

To Remove Detergent Residue

Washing Machine Cleaner

You'll need:
1 cup Epsom salt
4 cups vinegar
Hot water

Instructions:
1. Fill empty washing machine with hot water.
2. Add Epsom salt and vinegar.
3. Agitate washing machine for 1 minute.
4. Allow to stand to 1 hour.
5. Agitate again for 1 full wash and rinse cycle.

Bring Your Car Battery Back to Life

Lead Acid Battery Booster

You'll need:
Epsom salt
Distilled water, heated up to 66°C (150°F)

Instructions:
1. To heated distilled water, stir in Epsom salt until it no longer dissolves.
2. Pour solution into battery. The electrolyte level will rise, but do not remove it.
3. Do not overfill, and do not pour undissolved Epsom salt into the battery.
4. Charge or equalize the battery.
5. Treatment may take about a month before it works.

NOTE: This usually works with older battery models. Newer batteries have their own additives to prevent sulfate buildup.

Recipes for the Garden

By using Epsom salt, we can do our share in reducing the amount of destructive chemicals put in the soil or used for plants. Epsom salt has been used for centuries for planting and gardening. The magnesium in Epsom salt aids in chlorophyll production, nutrient uptake, and seed germination. Epsom salt makes your plants bigger and healthier! Fruits and vegetables of a plant that has been nourished with Epsom salt are bigger and more delicious.

For Plant and Soil Nourishment

Plant Supplement

You'll need:
1 tablespoon Epsom salt to every foot of plant's height

Instructions:
1. Sprinkle appropriate amount on soil around your plant once a week.
2. Good for roses, tomatoes, peppers, houseplants and flowering plants.

For Greener, Lusher Grass

Lawn Fertilizer

You'll need:
2 tablespoons Epsom salt for each gallon of water needed for watering

Instructions:
1. Dissolve in water or sprinkle over grass before watering with hose or sprinklers.
2. Best done in springtime.

To Remove Tree Stumps

Tree Stump Remover

You'll need:
Epsom salt
Water

Instructions:
1. Trim the stump.
2. Drill several holes (1 inch wide x 1 foot deep) into the tree stump.
3. Fill holes with Epsom salt.
4. Pour water into the holes as well.

5. If stump is close to the ground, covering with mulch will speed the process.
6. Watch for evaporation and replenish Epsom solution if needed.
7. The stump will begin to decay after a few weeks.

For Brightly Colored and Abundant Blooms

Flowering Aid

You'll need:
½ cup Epsom salt
1 gallon warm water

Instructions:
1. Dissolve Epsom salt in water.
2. After watering with plain water, follow with this solution, avoiding leaves.
3. Do this once a month.

Keep Your Garden Mosquito and Bug-Free

Mosquito Repellent

You'll need:
1/3 cup Epsom salt
1/3 cup mouthwash
1/3 cup beer

Instructions:
1. Mix thoroughly and place in spray bottle.
2. Spray yard or garden to repel mosquitoes.
3. Spray once a month or more frequently, if needed.
4. Avoid spraying flowering plants.

Bug Repellent

You'll need:
2 2/3 cups each Epsom salt, beer, and mouthwash
2/3 teaspoon yeast

Instructions:
1. Mix together in a spray bottle or any container with a lid.
2. Cover and shake mixture.
3. If needed, stir to dissolve Epson salt and yeast completely.
4. Spray yard and garden to repel insects.
5. Avoid spraying plants that have flowers.

An Eco-Friendly Way to Kill Weeds

Weed Killer

You'll need:
2 cups Epsom salt
1 gallon white vinegar
¼ cup dishwashing liquid

Instructions:
1. Combine and put into spray bottle.
2. Spray weeds every two weeks or as needed.

Get Rid of Slugs in Your Garden

Slug Deterrent

You'll need:
Epsom salt

Instructions:
1. Sprinkle Epsom salt wherever you see the slugs and they won't come back.

Recipes for Pets

Pets can benefit from the uses of Epsom salt as well! The FDA has regulated Epsom salt as "for humans only," and it should not be administered internally except by a vet. Nevertheless, there are some helpful remedies for animals using Epsom salt externally. Keep your pet clean, relaxed, happy, and well-groomed with these gentle and natural alternatives.

Relieve Your Pet's Itching

Itch Reliever for Dogs

You'll need:
1 tablespoon Epsom salt
6 cups water

Instructions:
1. Dissolve Epsom salt in water.
2. Apply on affected areas.
3. Leave on.
4. Rinse off, if desired.

NOTE: Although the residual concentration of Epsom salt on the coat is not very high, make sure your dog does not lick the solution off its coat. The laxative effect may not be well-tolerated.

For Soothing Dogs' Limps and Sprains

Epsom Bath for Dogs

You'll need:
½ cup Epsom salt
Warm water

Instructions:
1. Let dog soak in this bath twice a day.
2. You may also soak a cloth in the solution and apply as a compress.

Relieve Itch and Treat Abscessed Nail Beds in Cats and Dogs

Treatment for Nail and Paw Abscess

You'll need:
½ cup Epsom salt
1 gallon of water

Instructions:
1. Soak affected paw(s) in bath for 5-10 minutes.
2. Repeat 2-4 times a day.

To Tone and Condition Horse's Muscles, Soothe Pain and Soreness, and Whiten Coat

Epsom Bath for Horses

You'll need:
1 cup Epson salt
5 gallon bucket of hot water

Instructions:
1. Water should be a little warmer than what is comfortable for your hands.
2. Dissolve Epsom salt in water.
3. Soak a large towel in solution and squeeze excess.
4. Starting at the neck, spread the towel over horse until cool to the touch.
5. Repeat until horse's body has been covered 3 times.
6. Repeat 3 times a week.

Other Recipes

There are uses for Epsom salt even in the most unlikely places. Here are some fun and amazing ideas! You can keep your yard and garbage can raccoon-free, make some beautiful, frosty decors, and make your steps or decks slip-proof.

To Keep Raccoons Away

Raccoon Repellent

You'll need:
Epsom salt

Instructions:
1. Spread the Epsom salt around trash can or places where raccoons visit.
2. Replenish if needed (The Epsom salt may be washed away by rain.)

Create Realistic-Looking Frost on Your Window

Christmas Window Frosting 1

You'll need:
Epsom salt
Stale beer

Instructions:
1. Add Epsom salt to beer and stir.
2. Continue adding until Epsom salt no longer dissolves.
3. Spread on window with a sponge. Sweep sponge into arcs at the corners for a realistic finish.
4. Allow to dry.

Christmas Window Frosting 2

You'll need:
1 cup Epsom salt
1½ cups hot water
3 tablespoons liquid detergent (use white- or blue-colored liquid)

Instructions:
1. Stir Epsom salt and dishwashing liquid into hot water. Allow to cool down.
2. Spread on window with a sponge. Sweep sponge into arcs at the corners for a realistic finish.
3. Allow to dry.

Decorate Crafts with Frost-Like Crystals

Fake Snow and Frost for Crafts

You'll need:
Epsom salt
Craft glue

Instructions:
1. Spread glue over surface to be "frosted."
2. Sprinkle Epsom salt over glue.

Quick and Easy Way to Create Non-Slip Surfaces

Non-Slip Surface

You'll need:
Epsom salt
Fresh, wet paint

Instructions:
1. Paint areas that need to be slip-proof.
2. Sprinkle Epsom salt over wet paint to create a non-slip surface when dry.

56

Conclusion

Epsom salt is an unassuming, natural, and versatile mineral compound. It is just as effective whether it is plain without any frills or dressed up in luxurious oils and scents. It's one of the old traditions that is worth keeping alive. Epsom salt is simple, inexpensive, natural and healthful. It gives us a chance to take a break from our modern, fast-paced, stress-bombarded lifestyle as we soak in a comforting and nourishing bath that takes away all the aches, sores, and uptightness. I invite you to explore all the benefits you can get from Epsom salt and hope that you could also come up with your own potions, recipes, and remedies to share with the world!

More Books by Josephine Simon

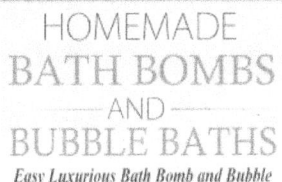
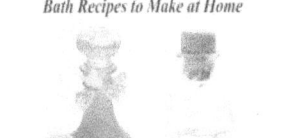
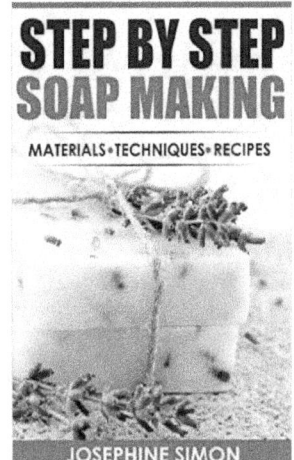
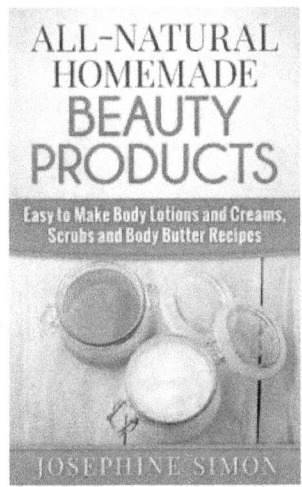
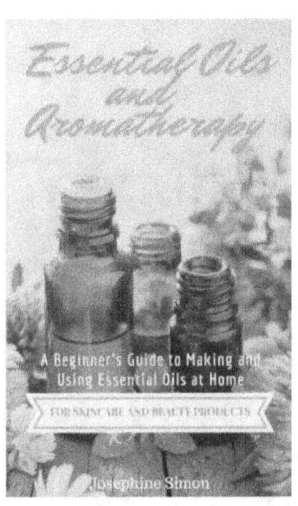
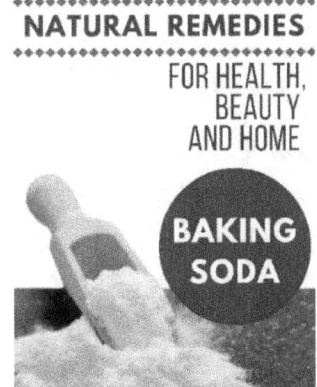
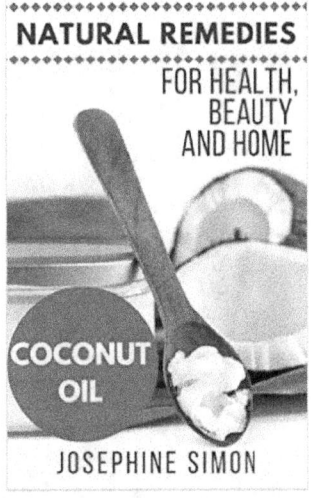
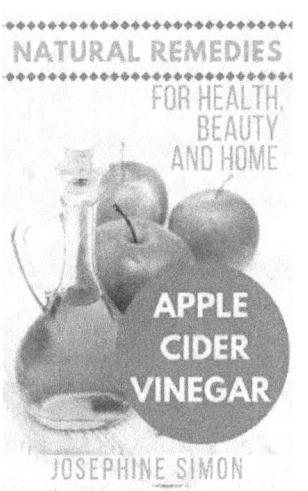